departures

departures

Dennis Cooley

TURNSTONE PRESS

departures

Turnstone Press
Artspace Building
206-100 Arthur Street
Winnipeg, MB
R3B 1H3 Canada
www.TurnstonePress.com

Turnstone Press gratefully acknowledges the assistance of the Canada Council for the Arts, the Manitoba Arts Council, the Government of Canada through the Canada Book Fund, and the Province of Manitoba through the Book Publishing Tax Credit and the Book Publisher Marketing Assistance Program.

Cover image: Shutterstock.com, Futurustic DNA, #268976129.

Printed and bound in Canada by Friesens for Turnstone Press.

Library and Archives Canada Cataloguing in Publication

Cooley, Dennis, 1944-, author
    Departures / Dennis Cooley.

Poems.
Issued in print and electronic formats.
ISBN 978-0-88801-563-1 (paperback).--ISBN 978-0-88801-564-8 (epub).--
ISBN 978-0-88801-565-5 (mobi)

    I. Title.

PS8555.O575D46 2016   C811'.54   C2016-901666-8
C2016-901667-6

to my family

departures

then, Winnipeg, hospital,
the Victoria, jumbled,
didn't know
where or when

they place him under the tree
he could be a present
could be a pheasant
sent to please   /appease

could well be tin
wrapped in tissue
tied in bright ribbons
could be a little thinner

could be a long marrow
an enormous sweet potato
smooth silver fruit
drinking the juices
the clear serum
could be a bat feeding
upside-down
the sweetness

because it does not hum where it turns
because it does not ring like glass
because it does not sound in diapason
because it does not want to let things stray
because it tries to bind all things
because it wants to gather them to music
because it blinds all creatures into believing
they might for a wisp of light slow the protein

it is not love but proportion
holds them together
keeps them from flying
            apart keeps them
            from having
                                to leave

yet of attraction what are we to speak
if it were not for repulsion
we would pass through empty space
pass right through one another
it is only repulsion lets us near

sounds drag over
throat through glottis
across tongue inside
cheeks over teeth
down nose out lips
consonants incisive & molar

flesh rubs vowels open
little blips lips add
flippant or whooing
lungs a periscope to our sonar

a hairiness too a brushing
dried grass over wood
the charity of unsaid wishes
voices spilled and memories
you, my mother and father, saying,
air you shaped

—᠆ᐱᐯ—

/it's science
a matter of pro and con
sequence & science
a matter of carbon & hydro
gen ox ygen & nit
rogen & a few others

that's how it is & that is
how it has been

continuous with us only in four
-letter alphabet "you can
take a fragment of human
genetic instruction, patch it
into a faulty yeast cell, and the yeast
cell will put it to work as if
it were its own" (Bill Bryson)
its simple codes coiling & uncoiling
in same & error & patently wrong
giving us the finger until it has
its way with us we ten
-digit two-footed ambulatories
with opposable thumbs and restless neurons
writes us off in its four-letter alphabets
and the cob of corn dwarfs us in genes

the impossible lines we are walking
a wide and dangerous globe
an almost legless Leakey travelled
4 1/2 million years all the way
home to Lake Natron we too

with swollen lobes in our heads
and dragging our genes behind

what then of synecdoche
what of
its measure the body's ailing
in whole or in part
what
it
is
to
be
of:

traces and echoes
speaking in echolalia
the relationship between
a part and a whole
the streaming atoms
the tangled genes
the of-ness of things
the if-ness

they say wind cannot dry it
fire cannot consume it
water cannot wet
nor earth rot

our days yes are fields
are as the fields of grass
we are made to lie down in
but to lie together in them
smell the crushed grain & flowers
the small dust of their perfume
fallen dust of the world

the sweet bundles of flesh
we have only now to touch

iron wheels roll
stonily across our lives
casters over ceramic floors
the sheets that cover the world
and some times warm

the horizon over which we are
carried seems roughly sewn
it is an issue one would think

the light stretched until it is
thinner than tissue
at times fibrous & torn
a spider's threads
sewing the four corners

throws us 1,000
miles per hour 24
hours a day we
do not fly off
nor do our eyes water
nor do we lose our feet
when we measure time
nor wind in our hair
not though we are hung
upside down
from the wobble
in the planet
do we feel dizzy

not even as the earth
hums all the way
there & back &
back again
hisses a round
the sun so
tipsy it
almost skips
out of the grooves
spins on/off
on/off on/off
painfully bright
in the dark soil

do not attend the rites or amend the wire
fences through which we hear
the world's music the wind
descend in frost-white ether
staple the window shut
                    press upon eyes

          you draw into
          untouched spaces
          your body at night
          listens to light

                    foot singing there's a ribbon
                    a ribbon of darkness

                    asleep dreaming
                    the carbon dioxide
                    stirs your sleep

We're going to show you what happened. His mother's voice, though she is dead. We have decided to show you what happened. To your aunt and grandmother. He knows no aunt, lost.

next day
        afternoon kitchen
        his mother rolling
        out a moon of dough
she will slide into an iron furnace
the kindling will crackle to crust

the machine grinds on, unfathomably slow, the wheel ponderous. **Hnnhhn-hnnnh-nhnn** lights roll heavily over. on his back in his grampa wilson's back yard, the wheel above him grinds on and on **hrrrhr–hrrhh–hnrh**. clock-wise. there is nothing he can do. it rolls on, laboriously, about to crush.

)he lies on his back. watches.

night so heavy he
can hardly
breathe
alongside the sagging & creaking

clock shudders & talks
in alarm talks
to itself
talks to him

he can hear
the shadows outside
drop from the window
fall in knots
onto his grampa's floor
feel them pool & clot

the hot stars
caught in their hair
are talking *click*
click *clickclick*
black angels all night
long on the other side
the porous curtains shift
the clock listens
through the dusty holes
watches

Begin Your Journey

Know who has been in your genes.

All this with our Secret Testing Methods. A toothbrush, wax from your ear, a hair from your leg, a follicle from your nose, a toenail, even your spit—in all these are the secrets of your Relatives kept.

Discover who is your Twin, your own Sibling.
Determine who is your Grandparent.
See if you are your Father.
Or your own Daughter.

All this for only $189.
ALL THIS AND MORE.

Simply swipe and send.

Just leave it to us.
Let's keep it in the family.

sun skids across the floor
well and fairly portioned
seemly it might be said

amorous where it swings
with the enormous moon
the glamorous stars
& sometimes rain
plunges down gutters & rain
pipes through the cold & dark

earth grates and heaves itself
through the swarming stars
gyrates on its armature
plunges & swoops so wild
the stomach falls out

it comes
down slowly

more heavy than
boulders, then
faster and faster

the trees crack and the branches begin
to fall

there aren't this many
in his grampa's yard
their branches breaking
shedding leaves

they know where
his fear began   they will
find it say they will
help him say.

old trees dying
they say redirect
their energies nudge
younger trees to
root & blossom

something he is supposed to reach & touch.
has killed an aunt he never knew, and his
grandmother. something,
under the roof or eaves.
he cannot move.

Look. There's the man in the moon.
His dad holds him up in his right arm.
Do you see the man in the moon?
No, he said, the small boy said, disappointed.
He could not see him.
He tried hard but he could not
see the man in the moon.

home from school over
the scabrous & cactused hill
the coal stove splintering heat into the kitchen

blaze of kindling
sun washing
the winter window
leaking weakly

his mother is rolling
a moon of dough

stoops and
/pops it
/into the oven

waits for it
to turn
copper
out of sight

world begun.
world undone.
the earth's rind grinds
down to grit down to
chaff & dust—

turns all the way, once. Could be months.
Years. Seems years. The lights rumble on & on & on—

and then
it be
gins to
descend

it is massive &
clumsy & it
begins to descend

and another time:
whhuuu-ummpmpp.
/they land
/hard

and then another
whhummpmpp

as in "the hum of distant traffic"

Rrhhrummm rhrhumm
hrrhuum rrhummp
rrhhrummm
Rhrhumm hrrhuum rrhummp

730 a.m. Thurs feb 22, he thinks it is

moved through the night on a bicycle
a kid's ccm without wheels
grasps the shiny frame and watches
a man and a big piece of clear plastic
        his hand dips
into a pail of vinegar he's been
polishing the moon
shining to brightness
so luminous his breath catches

—

the world veil spins
            around him tangles
his thoughts twist
            inside his head & out side
the skeins fold &
flop against the flow a
                        distant voice
distinct & unperturbed

sometimes talks about an area in the u.s.
a low forest around it and in it
            an abandoned baby stroller
a lot of garbage & cars passing

            the first skein
in the world or beginning
has been dumped here

the skeins cross other skeins
            dirty white or gray
            some of them renegade
some known only to him

—

the voice spoke with confidence
an exactitude that held him
it was low but utterly clear and
it explained the origins
the whorlings & gauzy clouds

the first time of the world it said the world
drifted over him it tugged & pulled

one line was good and there were
several lines that began the universe
the voice said and named them
the voice was official & undistracted

there were names for all of them and the voice
gave them   one by one

he got all of the names
pleased to hear them
though he could
not remember what they were called
and one of them
swirled off in a short neat spiral

he might have thought of the northern lights
when they cross the sky
but didn't
this one
was skirring and
utterly without colour

it was the genitive line the voice said
it was not directed to him
it spoke evenly of fact
talked to no one in particular, went on, as if
no one was listening

and it gave a long list of cognates
this was the line that included people it said
the line of humans,
hence the pre-fix "gen"

—

The other voice sounded like an old friend, dead now. Once he even called. Is that you Bud? But no one answered. One of the women sounded like Diane. He thought it was her, it was her there. The man talked & talked, people came & went, they talked and talked.

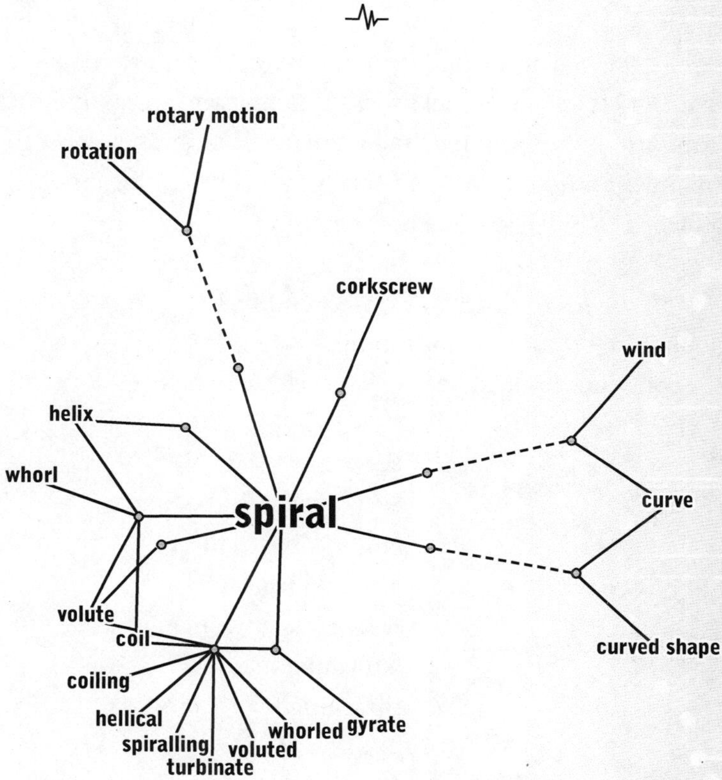
rotary motion
rotation
corkscrew
wind
helix
whorl
spiral
curve
volute
coil
curved shape
coiling
hellical
whorled
gyrate
spiralling
voluted
turbinate

stands over thin man jerks & twitches ribbons dangle from wrists and arms flicks flicks ribbons from wrists and arms arm man alarm man tall man on stick legs stick arms trembles for hours twists & beats his arms twitch the moon attached to his shoulder elbow wrist

bends in close   jerks and flails
above him beside   him at him
leans his stickness   close to the bed

stick man hit man
scythe man writhe man
chops & hacks the air
around his head
trick man sickle man
a trashing man
thrashing man

stick beating
air legs
arms elbows
loose & slashing
presses his face
nicks and clicks

pale man
frail man
flails the air
drags a moon
above & behind

shock man shook man
aspires to gesture
pines for motion
chops the air

-as if his life
-depended
-on it

it will get in the shadows
up & down the room
the graveldust the garage
the smell of gas and fishnets
the boarded light
the bamboo rods dip into

the souris
bright with frogs
he has impaled

& the wondrous slither of
jacks long as his arm
as spattered the day

The following table gives the chemical composition of a normal man weighing 150 pounds (from kellogg's new dietetics):

1. Oxygen-about 65% or 90 pounds.
2. Carbon-about 18% or 36 pounds.
3. Hydrogen-about 10% or 14 pounds.
4. Nitrogen-about 3% or 3 1/2 pounds.
5. Calcium-about 1.5% or 3 3/4 pounds.
6. Phosphorus-about 1% or 1.14 ounces.
7. Potassium-about 0.35% or 3 ounces.
8. Sulphur-about 0.25% or 3 ounces.
9. Sodium-about 0.15% or 21/2 ounces.
10. Chlorine-about 0.15% or 4 ounces.
11. Magnesium-about 0.05% or 1 1/2 ounces.
12. Iron-about 0.004% or 1/6 ounce.
13. Silicon-very minute amount, not even an ounce.
14. Fluorine-about 0.004%.
15. Iodine-very minute amount.
16. Manganese-accompanies iron in many tissues.

[it cannot grow by an inch or an ounce]

Would he cipher the numbers?
Or you, dear reader, will you count the days?

you dear
reader can pro
rate the numbers
for your self pro
rogue your time
of sitting

You might want to check the numbers.
You might wish to do this for cooley.
You might want to do this for yourself.

99.99% of all species gone kaput
wiped out & we wear the 4
,000,000 years on our wrists
because at the last
tick we always lucked out

catastrophes & fortuities side
-stepping accidents & misadventures
the multitudinous flukes & wrenchings
    we went through

    a billion doors
    a few thousand people
    sneak through at the last moment
    all that is left after the ice age
    sheer dumb luck
    we ducked under

    the whole lot of us
    that close to extinction
    that close to one another

disembar
kings the acro
bats disem
barkings
bar kings
barking up
the wrong tree

he wishes she would
bring him a bone
bring him a bone
bring him a bone
and take him home
bring him a bone
and take him home

Needles in his body his neck sewn in. A clear syringe.

Stapled shut. A bag of take-out.

Take him away
takehimaway.
Out of there.

Take-home the Brits would say.
He is a staple product.
Product of Canada.

You need to breathe hard, breathe hard and cough. You will fill up on water. You are not trying, you have to try harder.
He is filling up on ice they say, he is not trying.

And a young woman. Checking. Ms. Quality Control.
Ms. Staple.
He swaddled in bandage and distrust, a long angry slash.

Who is she? What is she to him, or him to her, she should peek at him? Would he be betraying C.? If he let her take a look?

you must
face the music
live while you can
keep your feet
live while you dance

in the end
she will leave you pale
rider pale ghost

when smoke from your mouth bursts
and on burnt feet you dance

The voice behind the curtain. Laughs, laughs. That will show them, all the shit they do. Wait'll they see this.

The voice has phoned, phoned. The voice calls and calls. A loud public voice. Can you get a truck over there? Can you drop off ...? The voice is making a movie. The nurses' voices tell the voice he's had a second heart attack—4:00 in the morning. He calls number after number, feverishly. The voice laughs and laughs, says it wants to go home. It wants to go home. It phones & phones.

That night, the night after the filming, more calls. Computers have searched out information on heart attacks and they feed it in. An assistant, somewhere, reports this information in a distinct voice. Cooley can hear everything she says about heart attacks. He worries about the man with the laugh who wants to go home.

A voice behind a curtain.

The laugh kicks
in and out
in and out.

/appendix

This patient presented with peritonitis
Secondary to an appendicitis on february 15th,
(on which day the moon had fully dilated)
1996, in Winnipeg manitoba. Laparotomy,
Appendectomy and drainage were required.

ruptured before he came in
his body soaked in toxins

A septic field he says, the anesthesiologist.
when he reappears.
a septic tank.

all the years they had
together and now
without warning or apology
it has
up & left him

which may induce in the skeptical
fears of contagion.
or incoherence.

you can read it in the stars
or, if you prefer, under the ribs
under the stairs DNA is wound
round a ladder
life climbs aboard is heir to
the bundle of proteins
that is you is me is us
over & over & over again
flagrant abuse against copyright
theft of private property not
to mention also damage

enough in one of us if it were to be
pulled like toffee would reach the moon
all the way to the man no one can see
and back and out and back and out and back
and out and back again

to the man in the moon
the queer old balloon man
on the end of a string
astringent with wish

itch man twitch man
waking man shaking man
yanks & jerks
coming & going
on a yo-yo
does not whistle
does not play

look his dad said
the man in the moon

genetics is we can agree
what most matters
to you is postmodern

there being dissonance
in such matters generally
it is generic of a kind unkindly

yet in gestation generous & in generation
plenty of noise in the system
stray chunks & trays of broken pieces
in odd places add
nothing it seems to the whole

no one knows what
it is doing there or what
it does it doesn't
do much of anything
as far as we can see
what good is it

a few strands
with no discernible purpose
or intelligible affect
and an awful lot of garbage

Per: it on

it is:

a person left hanging

It is in flammation of the peritoneum, the membrane lining the organs within the abdomen and the wall of the abdominal cavity. Peritonitis is classified as bacterial, chemical, or haemorrhagic, depending on the cause. Bacterial peritonitis can be caused by perforation of an infected organ, such as the appendix. Chemical peritonitis can be caused by chemicals released from the digestive tract, such as bile or stomach acids. Haemorrhagic peritonitis may be caused by a violent blow to the abdomen causing internal bleeding. Whatever the cause, peritonitis is a grave condition and usually requires surgical treatment and hospitalization.

ANDDNAANDDNAANDDNAANDDNAANDDNAANDDNA
ANDDNAANDDNAANDDNAANDDNAANDDNAANDDNA
ANDDNAANDDNAANDDNAANDDNAANDDNAANDDNA
ANDDNAANDDNAANDDNAANDDNAANDDNAANDDNA
ANDDNAANDDNAANDDNAANDDNAANDDNAANDDNA
ANDDNAANDDNAANDDNAANDDNAANDDNAANDDNA
ANDDNAANDDNAANDANDDNAANDDNAANDDNAAND
DNAANDDNAANDDNAANDDNAANDDNAANDDNAAND
DNAANDDNAANDDNAANDDNAANDDNAANDDNAAND
DNAANDDNA

and Megan
and Diane
and Dana

so also an an
a nada under
can ada among
the canaanites

known also as phoenicians
who found themselves lost
at sea at a loss for words

the shouts & whispers
the body vibrates
the illicit romance
every clasp and spasm
the endless chemical gossip
gabba gabba gabba
working the gaps
its small & inaudible gasps

psst ppstt presses the doors
in yeas & nays slamming
          /open and shut

speaks surprise & yearning
Heraclitus heard and knew
was the world spinning

its own high-wire act
which when there are
means & mess
engers hot little
engines aching
to make contact

their cupidity hard to refuse
or fault

their anger too
hard angles of that

knowing where they woo
at any & every synapse
arrive with messages that snap
the brain engenders danger

they are apt to be
spurned turned
away or off

a cool reception
the cold shoulder

if that be not enuff
yet always there is that
libertine carbon
dating everything in sight
everything it can lay

hands on or in
swapping will prove the life
of the party

which in taking
is taken without
which we would not be
much less any 4

,000,000 years for us
give or take a few
and counting

four very small cups. chicken broth.
cranberry, a thick sweet juice. the
smallest bit of each. flavour strong
and lingering. almost overpowering.
.5 grams
she reports.

Wild about Harry

The most famous person to die from a burst appendix was Harry Houdini, born Erich Weisz of Budapest. Dead at, yes, Hallowe'en. 1926. Houdini had prided himself on the strength of his pectoral muscles, modelled tight-fitting clothes. He put on quite the show. He had a real sense of theatre. You might think he was rather prissy but no, he challenged all comers to punch him, go ahead and slug him in the stomach, why don't they? Whack him a good one. He didn't feel a thing, they couldn't touch him. Nothing could phase him.

Some say the final blow, a Canadian in Montreal, killed him, exploded his appendix. Some say, no, that couldn't be, the appendix was already going.

Houdini himself believed someone for once had hurt him but he carried on through the pain. For years he had dazzled with his twists & squirms. He slipped locks, unstrung ropes, ripped off jackets, stripped chains, unlocked snaps and buckles; he sprung open padlocks and unshackled handcuffs. And the clocks ticked on. He plunged through boxes, leapt from tanks and water and sand, tipped like a bat upside down from a straight jacket slipped out. No prison could hold him. People got off on the peephole life, grew dizzy with excitement, they couldn't get enough. He led a charmed life, lacked nothing, such a handsome young man, so poised.

By the time they got him to the hospital it was too late. As luck would have it, there were no antibiotics to unfasten the poisons. There was no getting out of this one, you see, and he died from a massive infection he couldn't shake.

to be for getting out of time
be for getting out of time to
for getting out of time to be
getting out of time to be for
out of time to be for getting
of time to be for getting out
time to be for getting out of
to be for getting out of time

for seeking
for saking

all others
the world over
taking

—

Burning. A bright tower. She sits inside, waiting. The lights crack and pop, hundreds and hundreds of them. The tower creaks and detonates.

A long long time and then
finally it
goes down,
twists
on slow motion legs
and crumples.

a few people drift down a river. the front of a big plane, drifts, drifts. comfort, quiet. now and then in other parts, faint voices.

the arm a mess of scar and metal. No, Megan says, reaches over, we need this.

Yes, in another part of the boat. Yes they are fine, they'll be here soon.

She will say he meant his arm, or she thought
he meant his arm.

Yes, it's yours.

—

What day is it? Where is he? He doesn't know, doesn't know. Doesn't know when. Laughs at his mistakes, embarrassed and helpless. They can reach him at the University of Victoria. Victoria, they should send his mail to Victoria.

Don't know where. Didn't know when. Time in that bed, one spot, lost track of himself. Didn't know.

—∿—

sits at the end of the ward
at the end of the world
it is very cold

.winter squeezes
.through the windows
.at the end of the hall
.at the end of it all

february, his feet cold. always cold.

a horrendously distended stomach fastened to a machine
Sits in an orange robe
he will lose in Kraków.

Could be a squash growing from a pole.
Could be a pumpkin among dead vines.
Could be king of the gourds.

a long tuber
fatter than earth
no softer than
a white radish
a spaghetti squash
feeds from the shining tube
they hold him under
drop him from

would be a plant drinking from the window
the glass a shine of water
its cold clear wetness

he will die in the high cold night

—

man in spotted skin
shy and stunned or so he seems
his blue feet and rotten teeth his mouth
without sound his handsome
& bewildered face
sits in the hall with his family
and his stolen speech

—

skinny old geezers their watery gaze
weeds in a winter garden
raw-boned men who when they
bend could be leaking heat
when they bend squeezing
sniffs & wheezes

if you look where they are not
looking you see
fuzz & white buzzes of light
blend to wind & land

ribbed and ribboned
they sit in their grace
their shin bones glow
through the flannel
ironed by cold

the rafts of their bodies
they have almost left

    old men sticking it out
    on a windy ocean

—

It is not fibrous, there are no veins or threads. It is smooth but it is not shiny or slick. It glows it seems with its own light, light green to yellow, shape of a rootless molar. A gumdrop.

A phosphorescent gland, green and golden very deep he follows down, a big slough in Saskatchewan seven or eight feet deep. He can feel it pulse. He can almost see through it.

Another time an old computer, hot and smelling, in oil and huzz. It contains occult lore, formulae, health records.

—

scoops the water
knows it will heal

knows she is
watching knows she must

rescue him by the wrist
there is nothing

he can say or do no
way he can say

Let's go she says.

they infiltrate his camp
kill a worker just behind
the trailer they hide
the body in the room across from
paint the room over a man comes
out works his way sideways toward
wiping blood off

through the door a man
past his right shoulder behind him
walks through the door wiping
a screw driver
it is dripping blood
they have killed someone and now
they are coming for him

no no she says no one
will bother you here

of :

a pre-position : :

1) expressing the relationship between a part and a whole:

(one of these times, one of us)

2) expressing the relationship between a scale or measure and a value:

(99.99% of all species)

3) indicating an association between two entities, typically one of belonging:

(one of everything, all of ours)

4) expressing the relationship between a direction and a point of reference:

(1 mile west of yesterday, 1,690.34 kilometres to go before we sleep)

5) expressing the relationship between a general category and the thing being specified which belongs to such a category:

(a hurricane of scold)

6) indicating the relationship between a verb and an indirect object:

(to be of a mind)

7) indicating the material or substance constituting something:

(a morning of glass)

8) expressing time in relation to the following hour:

(a quarter of seven in the morning)

unprepossessing

Masked Ladies and Linened Gentlemen. A regatta of white sails look to the very heavens.

They wish to inspect entrails.

Some wait for wisdom. Some wait for a kiss. Some wait for ever. Some wait for Godot. Some once waited for Bardot. Everyone listens for the second coming.

At the Victoria they are waiting. The Royal Victorian Gasworks. And they will lean that way for ever.

And he—he, hero of this little melodrama, dear reader, surely you remember him—Cooley? He is no more to you than a municipal service? Is it his job to warm your homes? Warm your hearts with new-fueled dreams and scandal? The odd uplifting phoneme, a steady stutter of farts?

The Board needs something more.

It is an ill wind, he realizes, blows no good.

-∿-

out and music and they Over And the trace the Arc trace out after trace And then their swing, then sheer structure And rhrhumm They Over music the black and the arc another enormously another. angles. have after and angles. and swoop they bottomless. An huge have music they and rhrhumm rhythm. one structure they they **hrrhuum**. A rrhummp swoop Over they and rrhhrummm terrifying Over

a huge swing enormously and wonderfully magnified
the music of their repairs

5. To have the sensation of a humming noise; as, my head hums, — a pathological condition. [1913 webster]

The voice could be reporting on a budget, surprised they have been so cautious, there isn't much time, the places showing such strain. The thinking had been they would make a bolder move this time.

In the far corner his sister Lynn holds her course, quietly tends the threads that hold the neck of the harp they are tuning. She has worked without sound or light, unnoticed by those who orchestrate the large instrument, sweeping through the frozen aether.

a deep electric bass
drop themselves into darkness un
wind steel braids from their belts
sounds of plunging, a cavernous and frozen
dark they fall forever and alone into
might never come back.

WHAM

they maintain the broken hinge, fixing away. for 20,000 years they mend. there is no knowing if they can get it fastened.

the young men and women
ride their geometries skintight
glow dully inside a giant clock

Thursday 700 am

a gauze mask on the earth's face
the fields numb from sleeping
morning bleak with february

Cars drag themselves across the parking lot
nudge over sheets of dirty metal
clench against the cold.
All turn to face the same
way, watch through their
lights where they wait to enter.

Hunch against the wind, try to
keep their breath close, their
exhalations from freezing in the air.

Their lights spray onto the air
shove the cold through the glass
he watches through. The cold
presses him into the chair.

7 years for the body
to replace it
self completely new
except the same
old self everyone can tell
it's you & yet
it's not
you you are no longer you the same

things have changed and you are now not you
even though you are the same
bump where the finger broke
same slicing up & across
same long
boney feet same madness
for rhyme & pun same black
hair only grayer
you:
entirely different all the same

is it really you
you will say when i replaces me
where then will you be when
i get a new me & you you too
get a new me also a new you
how can i say i knew you
then we too who knew
who could believe are new again
who will we be when we are new

who knew you will say
who knew who could poss
ibly know or passably say
how we could know
one another now
and then

passes across the world
a sheet of piss-yellow
they tear & wrap
around bodies

long slow nights
every car pulls
the sheet up
yanks it
\down

untie him from the pod. a squid. a huge bean, fallen off
the beanstalk. a castor bean. castor oil. the tragical fruit.
oh do not cast your beans before you get them. do not cast
aspersions, neither cast ye kidney stones. the casting of. or
off.

*Castor oil is a vegetable oil derived from the castor
bean seed in its purest form. It is colorless, odorless
and tasteless. Cultivators of castor beans remove the
hull of the seed before pressing it to obtain the oil.*

Castor Oil for Skin
Castor Oil to Induce Labour
Castor Oil for Hair Growth
Castor Oil for Purgation

he is a has-been. a dead man. taken down.

They enact procedures. Reduce bandages, extract tubes. Ease
the hooks, unflesh lures and barbs. Cut off the brightness,
little by little lift him off. un-net him onto water. Leave the
knife in his side.

Complications. a cyst or tumour.
Rumours of lesions. roll him
and his mixed metaphors
on casters down the hall
to peer at his innards

C, 53?, almost shy,
reserved, calm.
M., 30?, sits
on the bed could be sitting
over coffee and what of coffee
beans she has seen

a dark spot she has seen
a shadow in the gut

demerol (*demurral* the computer urges;
also *demure*, and *dimmer*. And then, in polite reluctance,
or timely emphasis: *dement*). *demented.* is it rhyme
makes him think *demoralized*? a demon.
a demanding.

other adverse reactions include:
nervous system: euphoria, dysphoria, weakness, headache,
agitation, tremor, uncoordinated muscle movements (e.g.
muscle twitches, myoclonus), severe convulsions, sudden
hallucinations and disorientation, visual disturbances.

read more:
sEI ZuR eS, De$_{\text{li}}$

RIUM

FEE lingS of DISS O

Ciati ON

fRO M REa lITY

BLUR

RED OR DO

UBLE-VI SION ^{OR} OT

HER $_{\text{CHA}}$ NGES

IN VIS ion

LOSS OF APPETITE

Are you hungry? No,
no, i'm not hungry.
Thirsty yes. He longs
for a tall glass of
cold clear water.

nervousness or restlessness
Nightmares or disturbing dreams
unusual excitement or restlessness
(especially in children)

strong sense of rolling.
a trundling and he saw
windows on his left knew Diane has
brought him to Saskatchewan. last room,
two large windows, as they were
in the dream, and when he left.

every march every april
he could feel
the springs in his chest
the speed of the window
his heart rolled down
the loud wind

A bird, a large bird, long-tailed. It knows about this place, and with its long tail watches. Watches. The bird sits at the top of a huge tree without a trunk and long deliberate branches, many branches. He knows going up the tree to the bird he can learn what he once knew, needs to know.

They find out about the tree and they start. They poison the bird, and then the tree. They begin to rip off the branches. They wilt and fall back, and he cannot go up them anymore.

he had enjoyed the trip, and there were lanes and farms down heavily treed roads there in the tree, he could see and could go to and one day would.

I heard yesterday that you had a close shave with an undiagnosed ruptured appendix. For two days yet! I gather that it was nip and tuck for you for a while there.

Maudlin surely this
Is sentiment
ality in any event
you Al it tea
actually they
will say in to
Ron to or van
Couver & gal
Kerrie where they know
about alterity this garden
Stuff & Family
the same
Old rom
Antic past
Oral no
Thing to do
With re:
ality really

or in any event
the world
we invent
the one we write

he will be lying in a dusty parlour & a clock
spinning a house that never was a place Diane takes him
the pasture where the snakes had slithered

the wall calls clack
clock clack loud
& slow hour after
hour sour from not
moving he is home

sick for home at night
sick the clock
a loud mill inside
the metal night
his grampa winds
against sleeping

the wooden pipes
wait all night
stand like soldiers
shoulders straight
in the racks
never sleep

in the morning the
man with the milk that clinks
and the huge horse says
clock clock
clopp klopp

watch out watch out
here they come
here they come so
fast and big
he runs for the house

—

he had walked through his fear gone out of his way when
he saw the space swallow frogs whole slipping into and out
of gopher holes as he knew they would hundreds sipping
through the grass the shivery ribbons opening and engorging
more slippery than air and quick and chilled he had run
—

a garter snake sucks the world
down every night
a swollen frog
stuck in its throat
every morning a yellow
egg pops out of its black gullet
thirty days & thirty nights
the wet black ink
mouths wide-open
longer than night
we lie in our skins
do not hear one another
call out

& in the morning release
the yellow egg
bright spots of blood
running down our sides

But the bird. A perfect marvel—bird and garden. There, Frye tells us, we find "the identification of the human soul with a bird sitting in the branches of the tree of life." The tree in the weaving on the wall. The big and still bird he was seeing.

In the end they gain control of the tree. They mean to destroy the entire world. He can not say a word. There is nothing he can do. He lies very still.

at the end of
the line trussed & trestled

front to back
belly button to back
bone he had turned
10 with a broken collar
bone and they laid him on
the shoulder

left a red welt
as though ripped on barbwire
across his side
and later white

forty years later they slice him
top to bottom sternum to pubis

a pig strung up
wet guts spilling
bloop into the tub he is drawn
and quartered purple
& yellow guts a soft
sploop into the tub

in a white forest
from the tripod swinging
hanging for acts of freezing

the ribbons
red and blue and white
when he was 12 and 2
years after they cut him
at 10 in half

a picture his sister
Sharon claims still to have

10:30, one day, days later. Decades later.
She is on her way.

Sharon wrestles with the machine. Grips it with all her might,
letmego letmego, jams between it his face into
snow a fan blowing.

starts to cool on the edges, the air, a gentler sound, steadier, a wet coarse-snow air. march air. pushes toward the cool

"Wherefore is it that thou
dost ask after my name?"

Where are you?
What day is it?
Tuesday's child
is fair of face.
Who are you?

where is here?

one day Lorne and Laurel
standing by the bed

Something more is called for, some thing for which a gentleman would give his last farthing. Farting like an old dray horse would seem what's needed. It seems such a fair thing, in the end a far better thing, if he were to produce at least one single ting, a near or far ting. That would not be asking too much, surely. That would be perfectly reasonable.

Heads bowed, in solicitation prayerful, in genuflection solemn, in hope beseeching. A tingling. A tin ting, a tintinnabulation. That the pneuma might pass them over, and the spirit dwell among, they bend and peer, stand and listen. An elision in time, the world's lesions. Kyrie Eleison, morning noon and night time too.

All this have they done for him. How in the final analysis can he let them down? Has not he, like them, fallen out of the fiery comets and the storming gasses?

All they ask is a fart or two.
Are you hungry?
No, he isn't.

G., a burly man, huffles in, thick-sweatered. Seems faintly baffled. Hey, hi, pleased to see him, laughs when G. arrives to report. They're holding steady, steady as she goes. Waiting for gas.

They are expecting a break-through any day now, a new lease on life.
Time for release. And an appeasing of the gods.
Something in which to be exceedingly glad.
Something big.
Any day now.

Time to fizz. Time to fizzle.
time to break out.
time to break wind.

a lump of frozen dough, high in a cold Winnipeg sky.

he would stay as long as he could in the freezer summer a
blister his breath before him in goose bumps among the huge
carcasses hung from meat hooks you better come out his dad
would say

bodies thrashing on wind
& sometimes blown
off to the side
out of the way
in the end they pop
in awkward propinquity

We certify that Mr. Orin Cooley **died at Regina**
Saskatchewan on the 15th **day of** February **1980.**

(on which day the moon had fully dwindled)

ab-so-**lute**-ly
/zeer-OH!

beyond which there is nothing

a thermodynamic measure at which point
all motion stops it being
defined as a fraction of water
temperature which forms 6/10 of
our bodies that zero being 1
/273.16 of

also better known
    as -273.15
  °C and more
reassuringly -480
°F as can be verified
by the General Conference
    on Weights and Measures
      and can be used additionally
    to indicate levels of thermal noise

Megan. Near.
How will you get there?
There may be no room for you.
No, it's ok, I'll manage all right.

Diane in the back of
the plane, among the cargo.
He fears they will dump him
out. Come to this side he
says, here, to my left. Between
him and the door he means.

-⁄\\⁄-

He hates the dirt in the electrical clouds, an enormous old aluminum toaster, dust stuck on it. A pan, dry and pitted. low and gray, metallic. gritty hum. feels it on his hands.

Look at this. He brushes the rail and it comes off on his hands, thickly. old lace, a dirty powder.

She will take him away, takes him to a small room many floors up a tall thin building, walls lined with wood and gauze, a softer dust. The air starts to settle, slight smell of spice.

before that a mountain. hamilton, a steep climb, snarled with radio signals, music, voices, residues from broadcasting. a low crackly buzz, stations wrowling. a group singing an old collegiate anthem.

coffee shops with milk shakes, and then cinnamon and vanilla, nutmeg too, somewhere to the side when he'd come up the steep streets.

tea and spices cappuccino, powdery with chocolate, gritty
the spice-sniffers in their armadas and greed

in his own small room
he a small ship brushing
spices from the rail

The room moves up floor after floor a long gossamer furling and as he glides up it is piling up on him. To a fineness. A faint sweetness, powdered nutmeg or cinnamon, he is not sure, then or now, remembering. It is very soft and it winnows in skeins around him.

all the dust
you had dropt
when you left

The pill, a soft covering, faintly savoury, and so also is the water she gives to drink. More travelling up and down, breathtakingly long lines between buildings.

once they found
a frequency he could almost
hear bits
past the static
it was hard to reach
above and behind
his right ear the other side
of his brain the feel of the fan

it is february, 1995,
diane sets time and leaves it
there for him to read

boat on a dark ocean
whose sails might once have
creaked like crickets he
saw the harbour lights
steer him through nights
more slowly than rocks
weeks pass and the numbers
lie in red change smally—1:45, 1:46,
1:46—am it says am am am i am
you are we were
there there will be there once
more will have been everyone everywhere
the pronominal variance in our lives

chronometer of night
lights tuned to digits
as if he could dig its message up
a very small place
he could wash ashore

a small harbour
a wish
he could
raft /toward

told the time
time & time again
it was time
on the edge
he saw there
in the red digits

Like a madman. Looked like a madman.
A madman, madam.
Wild-eyed and staring.

rough ride on a macadam road—

be sure also to mention
the thick lobes light passes through
what once was part of Chaucer's beard
and a blue tea cup in Lyon, chipped
what has spent time in a flashlight
you lost in the park with a key to your office
the initials that were not his
carved into a grade-three desk
unfathomably deep & dead & enduring
the wooden handle on the hoe in her hand
and the keyboard plummeting
back into the sun

The voice sounded as if it came
through the nose it could have
been coming through an old megaphone
It was steady
                    and uninflected

      It didn't care
                    if you came.
      It didn't care
                    if you paid.
      Didn't care
                    if you said.

He is sleeping better they say.

Sshh she says
rest now she
says rest now.

"What happens really depends more
On the mood of the receptor than the
Willingness of the messenger."
Says Diane Ackerman.

he is a ribbon in a typewriter
the letters spooled
past the word press
clackety clack onto
the paper they leave
stains and wrinkles
spoiled you could say
or would have 30 yrs ago

consider : :

it is love calls us

to the body

in warm avowals

the sweet alchemy

makes and draws us

pro-position I:

those elements that in slip

page fall

together or cling

—Hy

drogen:

always on the verge

—Ox

ygen:

mild-mannered and quietly at

tending to see us

through and fill

with gas ready

to fan the flames

—these 2:every

"H" too

"H" to

/OH!

—HO!

the licking heat the crackling
fires oxygen so likes in love

—O2

it cannot resist holds nothing —O NO
back conspires in the burning
which is to say
its own consummation
its own prism of faith
hydrogenous erogenous
open-mouthed with vowels
the sheer genius of
ping- ponging
across the skinny
tissue of air

when you leave
will you
slip
under breath

leave me
where you bend
near
sleep
or wake
will you
slip your
arm from
under your breath)
falling back
into

under my breath
back into when
you love me

& when you leave
will you leave me
breathing will you
take my breath away

i.

if cooley's body were a little
less dormant if only he learned
the alphabet to tap the keys
on his computer integers
the enigmas buried in simple code
letters to be read and written
initials and monograms
found and known
on the way to revelation
a vision in steam
rising like a dream from coffee
from this our goodly earth

if he only showed a little
get up & go revealed a little
stick-to-it-ness tapped
the energy jammed
in his body he could come up with
some impressive results

if only he were willing
to do something for a change
deal with the half-life he's been leading
dormez vous dormez vous

it's a matter of energy they say
it could be quite a bit really
what it is he has in him that is
"enough to explode with the force of thirty
very large hydrogen bombs" as a matter
of fact if only he
would get the lead out

ii.

our atoms which know nothing
of us no nor do they care
one iota abandon us to court
the swampy & gaseous universe
utterly disloyal perfectly
ready to disport & frolic
sundown to sunup
gaily as they may
swarm the hot & honied cosmos
utterly prepared to fool
us fool around with any
old bit of fluff they happen upon

it's the same sad old story
¿isn't it

completely unabashed with starting
up all over again
with something else somebody new
whatever happens to flit by

and not a thought
                    at all of all
the days they spent
with you clinging closely
as ever atoms can for now and now
it's forget it who needs you
it's off for something new

iii.

no more promises of together forever
it's the same age-old shameless
promiscuity all over again
they're out there shambling &
looking for a little action
driven by promise & evasion
a life of inconstancy
the world in shambles

the gadabout molecules
          spinny with licence
                              break free
that's what happens with matter

iv.

matter in such matters enjoying
neither perspicacity nor
a particle of affection
for you or anyone for you
are passé old news your youth shattered
your dreams of ever-after bespattered
nothing you once believed solid

and you tossed
aside like an old sock
scattered like dry confetti
and the party's over
not long after the wedding

the watery pool cooley is
spooling into the same
old vaporous exhalations
and there's nothing left
    for him but
    a lot of lonely
    carbon dating

—

Sshh she says.

as if

he were
a coffee
cup

she wants
to cool

holds him
up in her arms

that's you she says
\points
|see
thats you
yes
/ there
thats you

see
//there
thats you

when he
waves
it reaches it
waves
back
it is

turned
around

puts his hand on
his face and the
other one puts his
other hand on
his other face

The strings in the world. Very long and made of metal, bigger than wires, girders almost—they are trying to fix. The ancients and Newton, is it?, are trying to figure it out. The world is running down, there isn't much time and they have to work hard. Some desperation. Not among the metaphysicians, they are quite calm. The rest are very anxious. Cooley too. He has forgotten if it is Newton, but he knows there is one Modern. They have strung and restrung the enormous scaffolding which is the world—an adjustment here, a testing there.

Repairs are not parts you replace,
they are parts you reposition.

no one speaks
they never speak
no net to catch
or surprise
no trophies for what they do

cat as trophes
cast as tropes
the disasters of
our lives so little
consequence to the stars
and soon not at all

once our bodies burn down
and we are feet squeezed
into the leather dark
into earth and the moon

is a stone
in our throats

we will turn with it
face all the other head
stones head first
in our bones

and the living will go on
herding up blood

& brooding

will talk and walk on

a gather of gravel
paths through the leather dark

rhapsody:

[Fr, r(h)apsodie < L.rhapsodia < Gr. rhapsoidis <rhapsoidos, one who strings songs together, reciter of epic poetry, a rap artist, rapt, rhaptien, to stitch together (, IE. *werp-, to twist, wind, whence WARP, WRAP, RAVEL, RAWP) + oidee, song (see ODE)], the twerp

1. a) in ancient Greece, a part of an epic poem suitable for a single uninterrupted recitation
b) a similar modern literary work

2. any X static or X travagantly N thews. I astic utterance in speech or giastic writing

3. great delight; ecstasy—hence X static, outside of oneself, beside one self, out of one's mind

4. (Obs.) a miscellany, Walt's yawp

5. in music an instrumental composition of free, irregular form, suggesting imp rovisation, given half a chance to rap but never wrap things up to let 'er rip in twisted letters let go with elastic news for the ages

the man inside, the paths
wandered .along walls. lost his way.
could not ,find his. way. back. the
end in his. hand, frayed, the end is at
hand. a burning, fuse he, follows his
confusion back. to where he .was.
before in time he ,remembered
and .picked .up the string,

She is turning in an ellipsis round the bed. He is to swing out to the very corner of the world and at the most precise moment connect with her.

her dark pubis swirling past again and again tilts up to
his right and he has to reach above up to her has to thrust
himself into her

> Gyration \gyra"tion\ (j[-i]r[=a]"sh[u^]n), n.
> 1. The act of turning or whirling, as around a fixed center; a circular or spiral motion; motion about an axis; rotation; revolution.

turning and turning in the widening gyre

Counter-clockwise in slanted orbit passes again and again. He has to get. there. If he doesn't, when he doesn't, he spins past or falls back. Gathers & hurls, trembles with the effort.

> It's just like a man, the voice says,
> justlike justlike.

it's all right she says it's all right they are dying all of them it's ok it's ok and he falls back the world is ending they will all die Diane too she leans over and touches—

There to the side.
the oval path

keeps us spinning at just the right
slant and motion. Delays in
the way the earth spins.
bulging at the equatorial middle
23 ½ degrees of leaning
drags the birds up and down the seasons
without which the earth would
fall off its tiltawhirl
shrink the tropics
to a narrow ribbon of emerald
squeeze the rest
into polar deep freeze

it's all right she says
it's ok   it's ok
hand on the back
light so light
it's ok   it's ok

can feel it leaving
where her hand moves
iron over washing
restoring linen to itself
it's ok

the windows of her skin
without speaking or asking
drain what has gone

the breeze picking up
smells of night

it's all right   all right
it is all right

bicycles, trying to make electricity, riding. everyone sick or weak, the room filled

    on the ends of lines, 3 or 4 in the room, big slings, what little they have, dripping into

what of the parabolas
and the cycles he found or saw
shining from moonlight
until they gleamed
amidst the garbage
and the one he rode
in spokes & rims

what of those he lay beneath
the mills whose noise ground
                    chaff and dust

what of those upings and downings
did the handlebars glimmer
did the music inside the radio
warm the dark
fields the red
numbers the half
life of things threatened with going
under ratios & trajectories

were they anything like the child
turning at the window turning & turning
everything churning everything going
a round & a round & a round
          or page's purple
sprockets the pedals locking
& unlocking the basement

the bed   this morning
swipes his hand &
the wrinkles

, ,

,

, vanish
under
the covers
her hands
he dreamt
moved over
skin

imagined he
saw her,
her hand sweep
across
saw it
splash & they

disappeared

little waves on water

know it was for you

i say to hell with the sun
it's only the sun

it's only going to take us with it
forget the goddamn moon & stars

rusting away in rain
i say seize the day

light squeeze thee three
table spoons into thy cup
drink before going

to bed hold thine
knees in expectancy

it is important not to
let on to feeling sad

know it was for you
all things were said

Is there any reason you might be well-suited to become an anesthetist?

Well, my uncle when he is talking can put a room full of people to sleep within 10 minutes.

-/\/-

The bottom of a depression, a skew in the ground. People come & go. His body washes off, or a part of it. He has been here before. He sluices through the pipes and channels, his insides, a swishing, quickness from site to site, slick fish.

Poisson. Poison.

To get out of prison.
To be released
in acts of misprision
pleased at last
to be out on parole
for given pard
oned which no one
can con done and no
one for old langue's
sake can do
with out
passing go

bends to the
sun the march air
coarse with half
-melting
washes off snow
flowers brighten
with light
bends to the
coarse air
sun with washes march half-
off snow
flowers with melting light

Ah Sun-flower! weary of time,
Who countest the steps of the Sun:
Seeking after that sweet golden clime
Where the travellers journey is done.

Where the Youth pined away with desire,
And the pale Virgin shrouded in snow:
Arise from their graves and aspire,
Where my Sun-flower wishes to go.

He lives at the bottom. For months & months, drifts down the small creek. Wooden chip, a catching & freeing, catching and letting go.

The raft is bigger than the creek.
The creek too small
for the raft. the raft snags
on the dirt and rocks and
debris and the waters
build & lift and
the raft nudges, regains
motion.

he would go back to the top again up past the small
waterfalls and the shifts on a sled he would go back
and it would gain buoyancy and then it would spin
slowly off down the cool water he liked the smell

a blue stone

for 4.7 billon years has swung
swoops round the sun
above or below
a huge gate we late
arrivals delayed by bad
weather measure in 365
days the precarious journey

outward and inward bound
summons birds to their streaming
north / south   south / north
the snows spread & recede
a blanket pulls over & off
pinches buds tugging
seeds in stem & leaf exploding
in bark & coo in verb & tangent
the blue & bearded earth

launches out and away flings back
pressed itself against gravity
that yanks it back
throws it
face-first & blinking
clatters against the raw light
near   far   around   again&again
an enormous tilt
or boom
erang

brought to an inch of
the man who lies
just over there
where he lays himself down to sleep
/by the windows
/levitating

above the bed
a hundred mill i
onth of a centi
meter the elect
rons run & click
particles refusing
any thing closer

the entire creation opposed to
further intimacy they are rivals in love
in what they call angstrom
what could be a swedish wrestler

an angst at the heart of matter
which /approached zips
/ off & away
that close but no closer

though what i am
when you are here
is not what i am once
you have gone

:

pro-position III

—these 2:

this at least is the thesis

- the story of
- theseus and ariadne

- add knee add love
- in copula above all

- a ball of thread
- a piece of string

- that is all
- that pulls us out

- all that holds
- us all together

the hardest things we do
knotting the ends into our selves
and an unbraiding of the self

learn to be empty
more empty than wind

lean into that
small loss of weight
that small wait

wait for me
we say wait
for me i can
hardly wait

A park. Diane has brought him into a park. A special wood. An american company owns the place. Tall grass everywhere, grace in moving, enhanced by whiskey—their whiskey, they say. And their whiskey is improved by the wood and the grass. They say.

sound of dried grass over wood
clarity of the unsaid.

he lies in the prairie.
in the cleft.
a shallow crease.
his body is turning into leather.
the edges of his body begin to curl.

he thinks he is dying.
he dies and dies and dies.
and he does die, once.

when Dana had been born
and he arrived from the long trip
heard her coming down the stairs opening
                    the door her
warmth pressed against

and when his grandmother
    died in the Christmas night
        sought him

i am not dead we are not dead her close silence said
        notdead notdead

and when he came back
from Germany cried
he was there

    and one time
from out of the place
where she kept herself
her sudden sobbing

        i don't want to die
        i don't want to die

yes i wld
if ever there
were

time enough or
room
i wld
lie

to you lie by you
lady
by my life
i wld

lie
till the last
crack of
doom

& after
noon & ever after

i was dead & died
every
after
moon & night

we wld lie
in several &
secret
places

when we are
good
& dead,

& the moon
is a bright
pan of blood

we lose they say
        exactly 24
grams at a time
at the exact time
of death the
precise weight of
    our breath
a time of waiting
we wet our breath

upon oceans of oxygen
smelts about to be caught
small welts in the air

no hope nope not even.
in the most cunning of moves
not though we are 2%

metal can there be a hair
        's breadth escape
        we cannot grow
by a gram or an ounce

certainly not when she passes
      or stands that
close you die again
& again for want of
wilt in your stale-dated body

and on baited
breath she takes
your breath away

Come on
back and
Take away

—

Days before somewhere under moose jaw a septic field had pulled him down past old lamp posts their heads hanging lightless streets barren and empty. Dana, he had said, and he had reached, when the threads wrapped him in their muscle. But he knew by then he would surface like a duck.

Now his body sinks, swishes water over, into. A grill, clogged. The minerals foam weakly. He begins on one side but as he moves toward the side he lies on, the sludge gets deeper and thicker.

Mud oozes in yellow and brown gunk collects in the pouches. Crud from the bottom of an old paint can. festering. anger. a vile stench. throat sounds, metal scrapings, broken loose.

knife at the edge of his ribs.

He sloshes water over pipes & plates under a bridge. Rinses out the stench

—

the wince when he does
& some times
falls back

who is to know   & who is to blame
your body   over mine shining
all the seas taking their own sweet time
making their way home at night

all the ups & downs
the self-love of the sick

—

Sags like wet snow. String beans when someone yanks the stake.

blister-hot summer
hose on full blast he tried
to smash grasshoppers
out of the rad. Water
and the smell of grasshoppers
broken pieces spraying
over his face

—

tending his splints, lifts the bandages, daubs softly. Her husband has just left her, she is alone. Leans over his distended and seeping body. The small sacks of mud. She is alone now and she is kind.

—

The air begins to shred. Sheds dust, sloughs husks. It breaks over him in small brittle husks. Onto him, sweepings from an elevator floor. Dry and itchy, worse than oat chaff on a hot august day, chaff stuck to his neck, his breathing.

Lights on dust to dust the edges of roaring you have to shout
you have to hold the noise from twisting your breath away to
death is close in august a furry man in goggles a snowfall a
fury of dust a halo of light the seeds pouring through augur
to truck rattly and then a deeper shushing (the sound of milk
in a pail filling

The man sits among strings. He is studying manuals. He is making delicate measurements. The lines, thin & oily, and the tiny electronic beads, also oily, need the finest precision. One or two nodules inside his head are out of position the man thinks and supposes he might find them. The man can turn one or two nodes end for end, move others slightly to one side or the other, front and back. Touches them carefully.

The tiny electrical bits spin & shine down long oily lines. The man is sometimes beside, sometimes inside, the computer, which is sometimes cooley himself and sometimes in him. The man is working on the gears and lines. The lines and nodes dangle inside, shine.

The oily gears, the ones in his side,
connect. The ones in the machine turn
the ones in his side.

The man sticks some thing in his mouth. Zaps. A foul smell. No, the man says, you don't have what killed my brother.

> This time he is inside, bending the tiniest bits, their intricate web. Radio whiz, knows the miniature bits, how to redo, and when that man is there there is the smell of oil.

Back & forth on a wire.
an abacus.
Birds on a wire fence.

—∿—

Longed for home, nostos.

remembered the story.
remembered home.

So did the guy
God breathed into
the guy's nostrils(horse
Charmer & he & she
Alive took his first
Breath the shock of that
a fistful of air
Nostrodamus lit on fire

Would you be willing

to donate an organ?

If so, which organ(s)?

Have you ever suffered from:?
(There are a lot of suffereds-from.)

Are there any reasons your organ(s) should not be used?

At the end of the long list of questions one
final one: Have you ever donated an organ before?

No, the woman writes, but once I donated a piano
to the church.

sometimes i can
almost hear you
further & further away
your body a broken furnace

can nearly
make you out
if it is you
if it is not

can't help thinking
being newly onely
it must be
dark & a little lonely

a little dark there
on the other side of the wall
the dark side of the moon

She talks in the dream he does not know is a dream that is not a dream.

::

so loud it is visible it has swirl and many
  forgettings between a future
                and a green roof
rocks too thin
too fine the dirt

he thinks green
fire thinks of her
a green fire when she wakes
when he is where they are

        her back
an escarpment he finds
hard to move keeps going
over vena cava venus all over
again against hope all
            over there
        hopehopehope
the sound of heliotrope

                    voice a salve
                a speaking at the door
                her somewhere voice
                hearing her
                a kind of healing

needs always to know
there can be no impunity
and who is where and what
are they doing there

body knows what is not self
it stands on guard for thee
alert to watchwords and shibboleths
identifies rogues (masked and
as they come and go (unasked
their acts of collusion & mutiny

asks of them passwords
ppsstt what's the word
signs of amity or old
acquaintance an instance
of good intention
or intelligible speech
give me the word
what is the world coming to

the need to sniff
out solecisms in halls
the stealth in small rooms
those who want to go over
cannot shush or speak admission
viruses feed & fester
befoul all sense of self
the closeness of contagion

body tries to set the locks on immunity
knows it is paranoia keeps it alive

Carry his body through the darkness, through the night. And there is a lovely old public building, brick. He has been here too. On the end of an enormous crane which pushes the room he lies in further and further into the sky, far out into the winter dark.

The room is run-down and hot.
a converted bus stop.
the clock on the wall.
he has been here before,
it is the same clock.

windows and water moving on up moving up in the world
will release him into the top of the stairs he will be out

there at the top of the stairs that are not there is a room full of
green plants firm with water, thick-lobed and waxy with light

the sun in his eyes
when he squints against
the woman who says smile
smile smile
for the light

smile she would put in a box
& carry away
his face in safe-keeping

meanwhile sun
behind him splashes
into a windshield

washes over his face
bleaches him to october
turns him into paper

smile for the light
in the light she took away
& the light that took her away

fleshy lobes
light passing
through & from

[There were no blossoms his memory says. Only the green, darker, and towards the centre a window on the edges, or everywhere, he cannot be sure. He thinks the leaves were lit all the way through.]

He will drink
the light and water.
In the next life
he will be a begonia.

Just now he lolls in a late-winter bin.
Musty old potato, white arms fumbling.

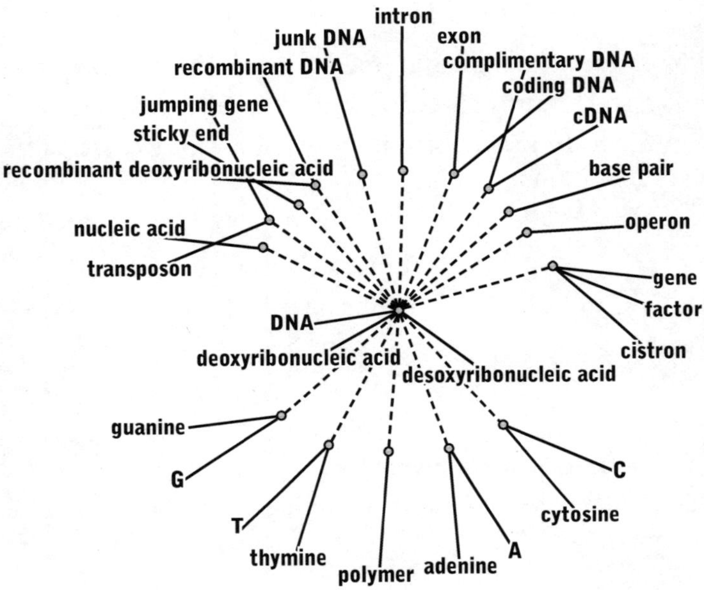
intron
junk DNA
exon
recombinant DNA
complimentary DNA
coding DNA
jumping gene
cDNA
sticky end
recombinant deoxyribonucleic acid
base pair
operon
nucleic acid
transposon
gene
factor
DNA
cistron
deoxyribonucleic acid
desoxyribonucleic acid
guanine
G
C
T
cytosine
thymine
A
polymer
adenine

leaves the radio with the silent man who called the
nurses when he climbed out of bed into
a hot dry room. Hat. Plopped. His father's,
herringbone, peak fastened with a snap.
buzzy junk. pitted aluminum. the dustpan shape of air.
Leaps from bed, in a rage.
Into his room, running.
Right there. It's right there. The plane. Crashed.
Press him to say.
He humiliated, angry—

unmasking man who had no visitors and now no left foot and
who called to help him. Nods, yes, thank you. for the sounds
that would be there he guessed. and the digits in the night.
radio releasing its small magic
into the dark

it is dark she says
Dana a little girl
at the window
looks out
the window evening
has entered
says into the gathering
it's dark and dark and dark

when you brush
thoughts sudden
current in an electric fence

leave a faint
bruise where
the sweet needle
went in

The poisons start to drain and the fever dims. the blur of demerol. Ground hog out of his shadow.

He is able to lie back into. The dreams begin to still. Begins to laugh in his sleep, talk with his friends.

He might be released.
He might go home.

—

Wakes him. Wakes him from dream. Wake up she says. The one who knows in her heart he is defective. Hurries in, happy to have caught him. She has got him dead to rights. Wake up Wake up.

She has identified him as a malingerer, arraigned him for weakness. A feckless man.

Justlikeaman. Justlikeaman. Hers a strange courting.

—

wish she understood
the way the wind blows
(wish i knew)
when you are bone tired
and she is too

Time to get up,
you better wake up,
you're beginning to talk.
To yourself.

A termagant. A harridan.
A hurricane of disapprovings.

Krankenhaus the germans call it

The hospital that is and this lady
Though not german
is certainly kranken
germ to his well-being
more than a little inhospitable

snip of mouth
slice of speech
her scissored talk

oh no no no
a pleasant dream
talking with a friend David
a friend's talk

✗✖✖✗

o now what now what
o now what has he done now

sugar in the morning
sugar in the evening

Big Blonde bustles in dispensing
judgments with a pharmaceutical zeal
✓ 2 each morning
✓ 3 at noon and
✓ 1 before bedtime
✓

the rounds of her displeasures
sounds of the world's but mostly his failures
regularly checks the cabinet of her displeasure
resolute to keep the dispensary full
and cooley on a proper regimen

It's no wonder you couldn't sleep,
What you've been through.

"nurse" : :

4 meaning(s) for "nurse"

1. (noun) one who is regularly employed to look after children
   - (synonym) nursemaid, nana, nurserymaid
   - (related) babysitter, sitter, chaperone, governess

2. (verb) to feed from the breast
   - (synonym) breast-feed, nourish, suckle
   - (related) bottle-feed

3. (verb) to promote the growth, development, or progress of
   - (synonym) cherish, cultivate, foster, nourish, nursle, nurture
   - (related) feed, advance, forward, further, promote, humor, indulge, pamper
   - (contrast) check, hold back, retard, slow

4. (verb) to attend to the wants and comforts of someone

- (synonym) minister to, care for, mother, serve, wait on
- (related) cure, heal, remedy, doctor, treat, pander

men are such sissies
she sez.

the indentations stand
night & day the lines slung
the blue cold the voices
                pole to pole
between which suns go
up & moons go down

along which a car roars &
        slides off wind
                        its swish

snow on the road
        scrolls open
                        & shut

          the poles rise
to exclamation sink
to periods that mark their passing

          the wind shoves
along the dark wound
          they follow
                    trying to keep
                                        inside the lines
all the way to winnipeg

his father back in estevan
                                    /dead

And what of this, then:
This story of ascent,
The halt and the lame,
The crippled, risen
Into motion?

Shakily writes. His hands swollen and weak, his eyes do not do what they did, thoughts drop away.

He tires easily.

In the mornings he sits in his orange housecoat in the chair by the glass a cold slab that shoulders into the room. His body hard and swollen. a tugboat broken from a frozen pond.

The heels of his hands are sore.

It is early march, it is bitterly cold. He writes these notes.

he tries
to write while
he can remember
what he remembers

His hands polished spoons. His vision changed. He holds the words like a censor—

Are you hungry? he said.

we were always beginning
and now we are
beginning to end
we are starting to end my lady
we are starting
to learn how
to end we are almost able
to know
how to end
i never knew
how to
say we are
starting to say
we are practising up to

stop do not say
this is all
we know
how to say
we are
here
& there
& there is
no other
life
not there
or here

i do not mean to be in
hospitable you know
i only mean
i never know
i do not know
how now (not) to begin

There's one other thing.
We took a spot
off your stomach, the long
spot on the first incision.

ribbon of
darkness

stain on the finest satin
a linen lace or silk
of which satan him
self would be proud

affection gray says
small fevers flare
that kind of strain
sunspots in the retina
empty spaces the kind of
grace melancholics wear

the curtain of his body
flaming with pigment
melanomas on the world's body
no one can constrain
a certain malady m'lady

it is melodrama
ends our lives
or melancholy
a shadow drawn
across the face of the moon

bella donna dilates a lady's eyes
first and foremost a prima donna
delivers into delirium
that portion that is
enough to keep
and take away

a melody in rain
a memory of if
if only
as if

The great bowel movement he supposed. A big shift in language. Fundamentally true perhaps. Good Canadian, he would say no, sorry. He should do better, didn't want to let them down, but no, he hadn't. No chance to air his grievances.

flatulence, hence of some
consequence of some influence flatulency
a fundamental fluency we might say
a basic speaking of under lying truths
a guest there in the body, a ghost that haunts us
a sudden gust, an inspiration, the gist of
listeners aghast with what is spoken
what secrets said to their face
a fart in the face of fate

a state of excessive gas in the
alimentary canal from whence it is
to be proclaimed if not concluded
for you too it is simply LMN
try my dear doctor C.
C. would get to
the bottom of things
if he played a hunch

the potential for diffusion
hence a propensity for
spreading the capacity to
amount to something
expansive in expression

home through the sharp february cold
home and he sleeps

I don't know what
i would have done.
They said you would
probably die.

& so

he has a religious experience
he bewilders himself

for 3 days he is amazed
where is it all going
where is it taking him

talk about inevitable
talk about ineffable
he has not eaten
for weeks & yet it
keeps coming his body keeps
turning it out resolute as weeds
in the cracks of a sidewalk

he who has learned
to doubt fun
damentalism
& now this that passeth under
standing

/sitting too

he is amazed he is puzzled
it seems to be using him
as it pleases the way it passes
like a weasel through a chicken coop
as if he were some vessel
holy shit he says as if it were given

on the way to rev
elation or at least elevation

And so it goes
Or so they say

he has got his wish
she has taken
his body sewn
shut she has
picked it up &
taken it home

He considers the contours of things,
the symmetry of chairs,
the misshapen body,
the roundness of water.

Cooley re-enters
the coiled and calling world
carries with him
a slashed and bulging stomach.
recalls Megan's own incisions.

Stirs in five-toed affection.
A tad slow, a low-lying
slow-breathing cloud. A sloth.
A little root-bound.
Moves with the ease of a rutabaga.
A flat-footed platypus trying to break out.

Follows the thread all the way out of the play pen.

Newly escaped and rotund.
Definitely rotund.
Definitely not Houdini.

his appendix
has up & left him
he will not miss it
not one little bit

two large patches of white
suddenly appear in his hair
one on each side

He makes plans for Germany —

acknowledgments:

Some of this material in earlier versions has appeared in *Sunfall* and in *Prairie Fire*.

Much of *departures* has been inspired by two brilliant books: Diane Ackerman's *An Alchemy of Mind*, and Bill Bryson's *A Short History of Nearly Everything*. In gratitude and waywardness I have drawn upon them.

With thanks for their part in the making of *departures* to Fred Wah, Sharon Caseburg, Michelle Palansky, Jamis Paulson, and Sarah Ens.

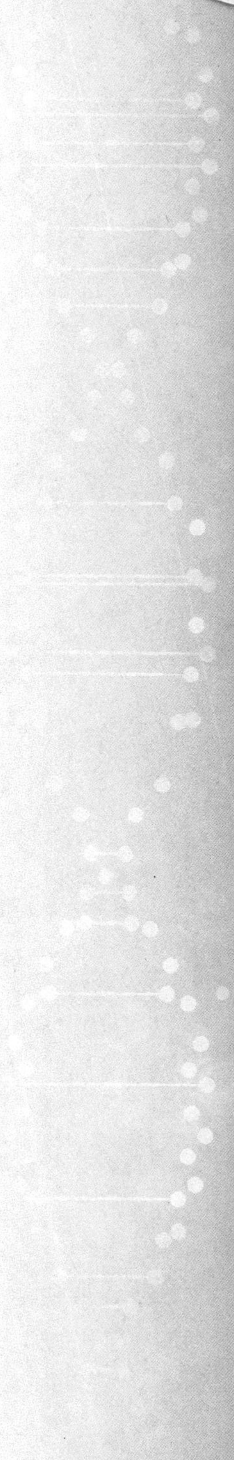